OK, IT'S MY TURN NOW

A DOCTOR'S JOURNEY THROUGH CANCER

DR. LAURA A. KATZ, MD

WAKEFIRE PRESS

OK, It's My Turn Now

A Doctor's Journey Through Cancer

Cover Design by Dee Dee Book Covers

Author Photos by Michael LaHote (Award-winning photographer and fellow cancer survivor)

ISBNs:

978-1-950476-31-2 (paperback)

978-1-950476-30-5 (eBook)

Published by:

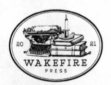

This book is dedicated with the deepest love and admiration to my "army." You know who you are, and I will never stop adoring you.

HI EVERYBODY. My name is Dr. Laura A. Katz. I am a fifty-one-year-old female ob-gyn in Monroe, Michigan. I have been practicing solo for the last twenty-plus years. I have been blessed and honored to care for thousands of women. I have delivered their babies, diagnosed and treated their cancers and gynecologic conditions, and helped them lead healthier lives. I have made it my mission to guide and empower as many people as I can for as long as I can. This little thing called cancer is not going to stop me. I want to be clear: this book in no way represents a substitute for medical advice or treatment. However, I am hopeful that if I talk you through my journey, it can help you through yours. Now, let's get cracking!

CHAPTER ONE

BICEPS TENDINITIS

THE YEAR 2020 was kind of a shit show for a lot of us, myself included. The pandemic was raging. The panic was raging. The anger was raging. Patients didn't know which way to turn. Fear and the media guided our every move. I was working in three different hospital systems, sometimes for thirty-six hours at a crack. Vaginas were deemed nonessential for a while and then, when they were essential again, no one wanted to come in anyway. So, it was kind of a mess. Diagnoses were delayed and women suffered. I was spending the majority of my time attempting to convert myself into a force of positivity unlike anything before seen on this earth. I was like, "C'mon! I am going to single-handedly uplift the spirits of everyone I know AND make sure that they stay healthy!" Oh yes. Motivational speeches, daily videos, the whole nine yards. I was loving every minute of it too. I still do.

In the meantime, I noticed that my right arm started hurting in September 2020, and it lasted for several months. I consulted with a doctor and was diagnosed with biceps tendinitis. I mean, it made sense. I was working a ton. I am right-handed. I always carry my ancient, non-lightweight computer in the crook of my right arm for twelve hours a day. I was doing a ton of aesthetic work and laser work with hundreds of repetitive arm motions. The diagnosis fit. Bring on the ice, the heat, the anti-inflammatories, and rest. Oh, wait! Rest? When is that going to happen?

The rest part didn't really happen, and the tendinitis didn't really get any better. I kept working because I wanted to and because I had to. My income had already taken a huge hit because of COVID, and my patients needed me. I decided to "rest" on the weekends. I was sure that would be enough.

CHAPTER TWO

TIME TO VISIT THE ER

LIFE CONTINUED, the pain in my arm continued, and it got more and more difficult to actually use it. This was, of course, unacceptable, but I was not sure what I could really do about it except stop working, which was not going to happen. I just kept dealing with it. I was fairly sure that my stomach had holes in it by now from all the Motrin I was gobbling. I was still bothered by the fact that my arm was not getting any better, and I started paying a little more attention to my body. I was starting to have some night sweats too. I chalked that up to being a menopausal woman, which was logical. I was also having a lot more fatigue. But I also wasn't sleeping well because of the night sweats and because I was working up to thirty-six hours at a time. So, I successfully explained that away too. I had more aches and pains, but I also suffered from chronic myofascial pain from old injuries, and that always got worse with stress. There was a lot of stress, so I thought that was explainable too. I worried about it enough to curbside consult some of my colleagues, but then explained my theories at the same time. Apparently, I was pretty convincing because nothing else happened or was recommended.

Fast forward a couple of weeks to December 12, 2020. I must warn you to brace yourself because what I am about to say will probably sound crazy. I was trying to sleep, in between sweating and aching, and I literally had a dream that I was yelling at myself to get my ass up and look in the mirror. I bolted upright and reoriented myself for a minute and then dutifully got up and looked in the mirror. Holy shit! I had a lump on the right side of my neck! Where in the hell did that come from? How long had it been there? I had a vague recollection of joking some weeks ago that I must have been really working out my right traps over my left because it seemed a little fuller, but I had let it go of course. As I stood and stared in the mirror, I got an undeniable feeling in the pit of my stomach that something was wrong. I mean, crap, there was a lump next to my neck. Was I turning into Quasimodo? I yelled for my poor husband to come and look. He stumbled into the bathroom and looked ... and saw nothing. I made him feel it. The more I looked at it, the more anxiety took over. I swore that it was pushing on my throat and choking me. That probably wasn't even possible anatomically, but I was convinced anyway.

I tried to get ahold of my doctor but wasn't successful. I admit, I was kind of panicking and felt like I was choking at this point, so my husband took me to the ER. I have to give them credit. They did everything right. They checked me over thoroughly. They made sure I wasn't actually choking.

Whew! They even did a CT scan, which didn't show anything, but, in hindsight, I think that is because it looked at an area a little below where my issue was. I was diagnosed with muscle overuse. Again, fair, since they didn't really find anything. I still left the ER worried.

CHAPTER THREE

I KNOW SOMETHING IS UP. I JUST CAN'T TELL YOU WHAT IT IS

POST ER VISIT, I still was worried over the weekend. I just couldn't let it go. I couldn't believe that there really wasn't anything on that scan. I know I have a stubborn streak, but I felt in my gut that something was wrong that we hadn't discovered yet. Now it was Monday, and I headed into the office with my lump, now feeling a little bigger. I decided to bite the bullet and have my sonographer scan me. Voila! We found a big, irregular-bordered, fluid-filled area right where I was hurting and where my lump was. Ah-ha! I was not crazy after all! But now, I was really scared and reassured and validated at the same time. We sent it off to the radiologist. I called my doctor, and she got me right in. She looked at everything, and we both agreed that we needed a repeat CT scan, only this time, target it more specifically to my neck and where my lump was. Unfortunately, no one could get me in for weeks.

Another week went by, the lump was getting bigger and more uncomfortable. I was feeling pain and pressure in more places. No CT slots were open yet, so I had my sonographer scan me again. This time it was bigger, and I could see lymph nodes in it. There were some spots in my chest just above my right breast too. Well crap! I had the advantage that I have read thousands of ultrasounds all over the body for the last twenty-plus years, so I had an idea of what I was looking at. I asked to be sent to a surgeon. He examined me thoroughly and thought that I had a lipoma, which is a benign fatty tumor. He also thought that it was pressing on other things which was causing my symptoms. He drew some labs and ordered a stat CT to try to get me in sooner than four weeks.

So, a repeat CT scan was done. Blam! There were nodes all over in my neck. Mind you, my scan was supposedly negative eight days before. I thought, *Oh crap!* But my doctors thought it was reassuring since it was growing so fast. It could mean that there was an inflammatory or infectious process involved. I was worried it was cancer. I got more CT scans which showed more nodes in my chest but nothing in my abdomen or pelvis. I was referred to ENT (ear, nose, and throat), who thought it could be reactionary or infectious too. Antibiotics were started. Now the differential diagnosis included infection, reaction, autoimmune, or possibly cancer. I wasn't convinced. Wouldn't I have been sicker if I'd had an infection affecting that many lymph nodes? I had enlarged lymph nodes in multiple lymph node chains in the neck, armpit, and chest: supraclavicular, cervical, mediastinal, paratracheal, and axillary. Usually, when that many nodes are affected, a person would be showing many more signs of systemic illness like chills, fever, and foul discharge, and they would visibly look ill on the outside as well.

So, I dutifully took my doxycycline and got terrible reflux

and crapped my brains out. By this time, I was having more night sweats, more fatigue, and more shortness of breath. Another week went by, and all the infection and autoimmune labs were essentially negative, except the one showing that I'd had Epstein Barr at some point in my life. I was feeling worse, and more nodes were popping up. I called my doctor and checked in. She said it was time for oncology. I agreed because, honestly, it was what I was worried about all along. She asked me if I wanted her to call or if I wanted to call. I made the call to the oncologist and was able to get an appointment that day. A diagnostic mammogram and breast ultrasound were ordered, and I was able to get them done right away. Fortunately, the mammogram was normal, so we weren't dealing with breast cancer. Whew! But the ultrasound was spectacularly ugly. Now I had even more nodes, and the fluid-filled area by my neck had kind of come together into one solid mass of matted lymph nodes, and everything had increased further in size. This all happened within one week! Well, that wasn't good. I never thought I would say something like this out loud but thank God I had an appointment with oncology that day.

The oncologist was amazing and very friendly. He took one look at my scans, examined me, and said, "Oh no. These are not nodes that enlarge because of infection. The nodes you have are pathologic until proven otherwise, and the size of them alone indicates that we must rule out cancer. This is most likely lymphoma." In less than one minute, I felt scared, validated, and weirdly relieved all at the same time. Of course, I was not jumping for joy that I possibly had cancer, but I felt like we were getting somewhere at last. We were going in the right direction. He said we needed a biopsy right away, and I wholeheartedly agreed. Then came the next snag. The doctor they wanted to do my biopsy couldn't fit me in for a couple of weeks because they were behind. No! This needs to be done like, yesterday, right? Even though the doctor assured me that two weeks was not going to make a difference, I still wanted to freak out. Two weeks seemed like forever at that moment. I couldn't work with how I felt. What was I going to do about my patients?

My doctor encouraged me to ask if it could be done any sooner. I was mortified. Did she mean use my connections? Did she want me to ask for a favor? I panicked and worried that they would think I was being rude, or that I thought I was more important than any other patient. Just to be clear, I don't think that way. She gently replied that it didn't hurt to ask and pointed out that I was not just asking for me, but for the thousands of patients that I needed to be healthy for. I went ahead and bit my lip and asked. Fortunately, my panic was for nothing. My oncologist had already found an alternative date on my behalf. I was incredibly blessed and fortunate that I was able to get in to see a different physician the next day for a biopsy! I felt like I had won the lotto.

CHAPTER FOUR

TIME FOR THE BEBOPSY

THE BIG DAY ARRIVED, and my husband and I jumped in the car and started out hours before the butt crack of dawn. A winter weather storm warning was in full effect, but we were determined to get there come hell or high water. I wasn't going to let anything get between me and those biopsy needles! I am not afraid of needles. I have multiple tattoos in different places. I mean, none of them required super long needles going behind my clavicle adjacent to my neck to harvest a deep tissue sample or anything, but you get what I am saying. There is nothing more ironic than the patient who comes to my office covered in ink and then passes out during a blood draw with a tiny butterfly needle.

We arrived at the doctor's office safely and checked in. Full COVID screening and security were in effect. Temperatures were taken and screening questions were asked. I never fully know how to answer some of them anymore. Is there any chance you were exposed to COVID in the last fourteen days? Well, sure there is because I work at three different hospital systems. There is a chance every day. Do you have any cough, shortness of breath, or fever? In this case I do, but it is likely from my lymphoma, not from COVID. I answered no anyway. I admit it. We were able to get in, and the doctor was waiting for us. He was great. He had a whole ultrasound-guided biopsy set up with a pathology microscope right in the room. The scientist in me was immediately curious. I wanted to look into the microscope too. I wanted to see my own cells displayed at high magnification and see if I could reach back to my pathology knowledge banks from medical school and help diagnose myself. For a minute, I allowed my clinical curiosity to take over, and I was almost looking forward to whatever we might find. Then, reality set in and I got nervous. This was really happening. I was really the patient this time. I was about to be biopsied for cancer. I started sweating through my Star Wars shirt. I had picked Star Wars hoping against hope that the Force would somehow soften the blow or protect me in some way. It seemed like a good idea at the time.

We got right to work. He explained everything that he was going to do and what he was looking for. We fired up the ultrasound machine. I cracked a couple of jokes to break the ice, for myself mostly.

He looked at my hump and immediately said, "Well, I don't like that." For lack of anything better to say, I said, "Me either." Then the conversation went something like this.

Him: "That's not normal."

Me: "Yup."

Him: "That's a lot of matted nodes."

Me: "I know."

Him: "Well, we should be able to get a good sample and then we can look at it right here for a preliminary."

Me: "Hallelujah."

And then he laughed. Then he numbed my skin, and I felt like my right boob disappeared entirely. He assured me that was normal. We got a bunch of core samples of a particularly angry node. I have to say, there is no feeling quite like the deep ache of a core biopsy needle. It's not a sharp pain, per se, but that deep, twingy, achy sensation can really make you queasy for a second. I think part of it is that you realize what is going on, and it doesn't match the feeling that you think you should have. So, your brain just improvises. Anyway, we got our samples and looked at them under the microscope. The first thing he said was, "It doesn't look metastatic." Halle-frickin-lujah! This is important because sometimes the really evil abdominal cancers, like pancreatic, can present with lymph nodes up in the neck. So yay, not metastatic. Initial impression: lymphoma, possible Hodgkin's. I actually got to look. Sure enough, there were a couple of possible Reed-Sternberg cells on the slide. Reed-Sternberg cells, also known as lacunar histiocytes, are giant cells that you can see on microscopy in patients that have Hodgkin's lymphoma. They are sometimes also called popcorn or owl's eye cells. These nicknames are appropriate because these cells have either multiple nuclei (cell centers), which make them look like a piece of popcorn, or just two nuclei with dark centers that look like a pair of owl's eyes. He would have to run the rest of the samples for official testing, but that was the initial read.

So, let me fill you in on Hodgkin's Lymphoma. If you have to get a type of cancer, apparently this is the one to get. Yes, it may require chemotherapy and radiation, and sometimes bone marrow transplants. But the five-year survival rate is a kickass above-ninety percent. Yes! I am going to root for that one!

CHAPTER FIVE

THE BIG WAIT

NOW THAT WE know I have lymphoma, we just have to determine the type. Again, there were a million different feelings going through my mind. I was scared shitless. I felt weirdly validated. I was relieved that someone believed me and that all these weird symptoms were not just in my head. That sounds ridiculous to say out loud, but one of the biggest challenges patients face when there is a diagnosis that is not readily visible is lack of validation. In the grand scheme of things, validation is not everything, but I honestly believe that it impacts a patient's health and capability of recovery. For me that day, it was important. I had felt guilty asking if I could get a biopsy sooner or see a doctor sooner. I knew in my gut that something was wrong and couldn't let it go. I also knew that this wasn't just about my life. It was about the thousands of women that I take care of. I had to advocate more for myself.

The initial adrenaline surge peaked at the biopsy visit. I was grateful that things were moving forward. I felt like we were making progress. I felt like I could actually breathe for a minute. And then it hit me ... Now, the next big wait is upon me. OMG another wait? There is so much more to do before I can even begin treatment! Doesn't everybody realize how urgent this is? I started to hyperventilate a bit just thinking about waiting for the final results. Then I had to tell myself to *slow down!* My inner rational voice had to take over. "Hey moron! Of course, they realize this is urgent! Um, don't you want them to know the specific type of cancer before they treat it?" Fortunately, I listened to my inner voice and forced myself to calm down before I made a fool of myself. Whew!

I spent the rest of the day being purposefully chipper and upbeat for everyone else but me. I tried to hide the fact that I was feeling sick. I tried to hide the fact that I was scared. I went into full-on badass mode. The possibility of having cancer somehow accelerated and heightened my sense of duty to others. I couldn't let anyone know that I actually felt terrible, achy, fatigued, exhausted, and in pain. I couldn't let anyone peek past my Wonder Woman outer shell. I had to be strong for my family, my patients, and my staff. They needed me. This diagnosis was going to potentially impact thousands of people along the way. Talk about self-induced pressure! At that moment, I became determined to make cancer "my bitch" and turn this experience into a teachable moment. I truly believed that I was meant to go through this so that I could lead others through it later. There was no time to waste. I had to strike while my energy was high and the iron was hot. I made a ton of plans. I had initially decided to try to keep everything a secret. I quickly realized through the advice of a wise friend that this plan was impossible. What was I going to say when I showed up to work bald one day?

Oops, by the way, I have cancer? That plan was a bust from the start. How was I going to lead if I gave no one anything to follow? In addition, employing secrecy would be like cutting off my support army at the knees before they ever had a chance to help.

I finally came clean with my diagnosis to the public. I vowed to write a book and donate some of the proceeds to the Leukemia & Lymphoma Society. I started my video series #imgonnalicklymphoma. It was go, go, go all day. On top of that, it was New Year's Eve, and I felt like the pressure was on to send out 2020 with a bang. Suddenly I went from planning my quiet, thankful, grateful-sigh type of exit to joining the masses in a big two middle fingers up to 2020. I realized that much bigger obstacles were waiting for me in 2021.

Then, it all came crashing down. After I made my diagnosis public, a flood of support came pouring in. This was amazing and heartwarming and overwhelming at the same time. Tons of people came forward to offer prayers, positivity, and good vibes. The patients seemed to appreciate the transparency. People offered to help and make food. The fact that I was willing to share my vulnerability with humor and a mostly positive attitude was like a beacon for everyone around me. People said I was an inspiration! It was empowering! I felt like I really was making a difference by sharing my story as it unfolded. I kept going all day. I was invincible! I was sure I was going to beat this! I was riding the positivity wave. And then, I actually stopped moving for a minute and dared to sit down. It was all over. My mind started racing in a negative way. I started getting scared. I started getting resentful. I was pissed! How was this fair? Why was this happening to me? Was I going to die? Finally, good things were starting to happen again in 2020 with my business, with my family, and with life in general ... and then I get cancer? What the hell? Did I piss off the universe? This is complete bullshit!

I started having a panic attack. My heart was racing. I thought it was going to pound out of my chest. The room suddenly got incredibly small, and I felt claustrophobic in my own body. I couldn't see straight. I felt like I had to physically move to make it go away. I somehow thought that if I started moving, I could physically move away from the attack itself. It was the only thing that I could think of to do. I started pacing around my kitchen with my poor husband staring at me helplessly. He knew he couldn't stop my runaway train now. He had to stay out of the way and just let me pace. I paced around, panting, for what seemed like forever, every now and then looking at his face. At that moment, his face registered a kind of sadness and desperation that I had never seen before. He told me later that I had broken his heart for the first time that day because he knew that this was only the first of many things that he would not be able to fix for me from that point on. After I finally stopped pacing, I plopped on the couch and began wallowing. I took stock of all my symptoms and began beating myself up that I didn't speak up soon enough. I turned on the self-blame and the pity channels full blast. This went on for a little bit until my brother-in-law called to check on us. He wanted to see how we were doing. For a blissful hour, I cleverly rotated the conversation to how *he* was doing, and everything melted away about cancer, and I was able to just concentrate on him. It was a nice reprieve. But it was only temporary.

CHAPTER SIX

WELL, THAT WAS A STUPID THING TO DO

MY POOR GIRLS. I looked at my daughters, and my heart hurt. I knew they were trying to hide their feelings. Kate was trying to be coldly logical, and Maggie was just trying to keep from crying. I felt guilty because I knew that they were already starting to miss out on things because of me, as if they haven't missed enough with all this pandemic crap. I kept trying to push them toward life as usual, but I knew they were having trouble with it. Of course, I realized that life couldn't be completely normal for a while, but I wanted to at least give it a shot.

You know what happens when people hear that you have cancer? Suddenly you become transformed into some sort of fragile china doll in their minds, and I hated it. I understood that I couldn't do all the same things at the moment, but I didn't need a babysitter ... at least not all the time. I wanted that perfect blend of sympathy when I wanted it and freedom when I didn't. The reality was that I just had to be more careful, especially during chemo and radiation. Yes, yes,

I know. How I got myself into trouble was letting my resentment of that reality get in the way of my common sense. I am going to confess and share a story to demonstrate just how stupid and potentially dangerous this can be.

One dreary day, I decided to go to the barn with my daughters. You see, we have a lot of amazing animals. We have horses, mini horses, and llamas, in addition to our home menagerie. I love them all with my whole heart, and I love the look on my daughters' faces when they spend time with them. They have brought a whole new level of joy to our lives. So, I was out there, and my daughters got the amazing idea to let me ride that day. They knew that I had been dying to get back on a horse ever since they started riding. I hadn't been on a horse regularly in over forty years, but that didn't even register on my radar at the moment. They tried to make it as safe as possible. They planned to let me just sit on his back, and they would lead me around, holding on the entire time. We were going to walk only. It was one of the greatest days of my life. I felt like I was on top of the world. I had not been on a horse in so long. The feeling was tremendous. I had finally stopped just being a bystander in the barn. I was so happy I could have cried. I was so grateful. My daughters were grinning ear to ear. It was a great moment.

And then, disaster struck. Suddenly, the horse spooked at who-the-hell-knows-what and flung me off him. Fortunately, I remembered everything my daughters told me in those few seconds. I tucked my arms. I tried to roll. I jerked my feet out of the stirrups immediately. I smacked on the ground with the wind knocked out of me. My daughter came rushing over and asked if I was okay. I yelled no, which ironically meant that I was, in fact, okay. The wind was knocked out of me, and my thigh was on fire. Thank God, nothing was broken. I was in pain, for sure, but I was okay. My first thoughts were that my husband was going to be furious. I was worried that he was going to yell at the girls. Never mind that I could have seriously hurt myself and held up my treatment. I worried about everybody else but me. It was kind of ridiculous. He was right. I should have known better. That was a stupid thing to do. I just wanted the girls to be happy and feel like everything was normal for a minute. I wasn't using my common sense, and I almost paid dearly for it. The lesson here is don't do it people! Don't get so stubborn to show people that everything is okay that you do something stupid. What if I had broken my neck, or worse? What would that have proven? Absolutely nothing. That's what. The story would have ended there. There would have been no treatment, and there would have been no me to be around to enjoy any more days. Lesson learned.

CHAPTER SEVEN

BACK IN THE HOSPITAL

THE DAY after my lovely ride, things took a turn for the crapper. I got out of bed victorious and determined to take a shower. That was my big plan for the day. This was going to be a good day! Well, I took that shower, washed my hair and everything ... even combed it! Then something started chewing away at my energy. I got a little wave of fatigue just getting dressed, and by the time I made my way out of my bedroom and to my kitchen, I was out of breath and barely able to move. But it wasn't really that I was out of breath. I was so exhausted that it was an extreme effort to do anything. I knew that I was capable of taking a full breath, but I just didn't have the energy to do it. I was so, so tired that I just wanted to shut my eyes. Something was happening, but I didn't know what it was. I barely made it back to my bedroom. I told my husband that something was wrong, but I could barely make it through the sentence. I felt like I was fading away. He decided to take me to the ER. I felt so weak that my daughter and husband had to help me into the car. Apparently, I passed out on the way to the ER, so my poor husband had to call a code, and staff came running to get me onto a stretcher. I came to on my own, thank goodness. I think I could hear everybody getting excited around me, but I just couldn't answer. They checked me all over. Fortunately, I didn't have a blood clot. My labs were okay. It didn't look like my cancer had significantly spread on my scan. Whew! They gave me some fluids which sort of helped for a minute, then the exhaustion washed over me all over again, and I could barely keep my eyes open. The doctors were concerned. It was time to transfer me to another hospital and get things rolling a little faster toward treatment. We needed to get me treated ASAP! I was going downhill faster than I should be.

An ambulance ride later, I was at the other hospital. Lots of tests later, no specific explanation for how I was feeling was to be found. Ah crap! No answers. I was able to get my pre-chemo testing done, so that was a plus. In the meantime, I slowly started feeling better on my own. As it turned out, we couldn't get chemo started any earlier because my final pathology report was not back yet. There would be no port scheduled this visit, and no insurance would cover in-patient chemo anyway. So much for that plan. So, what was I doing in here? Oh yeah, I passed out and felt like crap, and it was requiring an exorbitant amount of energy just to move and breathe. That's right. I needed to remember the line between advocating for myself and trying to be my own doctor. I started to waste time being frustrated and then I had to stop myself. I gave myself a much-needed reminder that yes, it *was* a good idea to know the exact type of lymphoma before trying to start treatment. No, it was *not* a good idea to put in a port before making sure that was the best way to go. I needed to sit back and listen. These doctors know what they are talking about. They have been doing this for over twenty years just like I've been doing what I've been doing for twenty-five years.

Meanwhile during my strides toward patience, I continued to feel better. I got a lot of time to think while I was alone in the hospital. Boy, it was lonely as a patient then. With all the pandemic stipulations and precautions, no one was allowed to visit you in the hospital unless they knew you were dying. So, I guess that was a point in my favor that I was not allowed visitors. It didn't make it any easier though. You had so much time to overthink, be scared, and perseverate. All the Skype, phone, and Zoom technology in the world did not make up for real human contact and comfort. I honestly think that the negative impact of the pandemic on patient care has been monumental. Patient family support has been study-proven to positively impact patient recovery, and we have single-handedly wiped that out. I have always believed that laughter is some of the best medicine. I can tell you right now that there was no laughter on these wards of lonely patients. I bet that when we look back on this years later, we are going to find that recovery rates dropped significantly.

Sorry, I couldn't help myself there. Let me climb off my soapbox and get back to the story. The tests piled up, and I continued to get better and was allowed to go home. I was going home with no answers as to what happened, and I had to accept it. This was not the same thing as being okay with it, but I had to accept it. There were going to be good days and bad days with this journey. I would not always get the answers that I so desperately sought. I felt better. There was nothing more to do in the hospital. It was time to go home.

CHAPTER EIGHT

GET TO THE MEAT

AFTER WHAT SEEMED LIKE AN ETERNITY, the fine-needle biopsy results came back. The pathologist called me personally, which I thought was awesome until I realized that he was calling to say that not all the stains were definitive. I needed another biopsy, this time a surgical one. Now he thought that my differential diagnosis included both Hodgkin's (the good one) and Diffuse Large B-Cell Non-Hodgkin's (aggressive, not so good, but also treatable). Yay! Ugh! Now what? Huh? To make matters more ridiculous, I started worrying irrationally. What if it wasn't lymphoma at all? What if I worried everybody for nothing? This should *not* have been my primary concern, but as I already mentioned a while ago, I have this thing about crying wolf or bothering people for nothing, I am fantastic at self-inflicted guilt, and I worry about drawing too much attention to myself. So, I asked the doctor straight out: Is there any chance that this is not a malignancy? He said, "No. This is grossly abnormal. It is a malignancy. We are doing the right thing. I just want to be sure about the type so that you get the right treatment." Well okay then.

So now we needed to get me to the surgeon for an excisional biopsy. I knew this was coming. It was what I was hoping for when this process first started. An excisional biopsy is a procedure during which the surgeon makes an incision in the skin and removes a sample of diseased tissue that is then sent for biopsy and staining of cells to determine what the disease is. Fortunately, I was able to get in to see a surgeon in the next two days ... and he was able to fit me in the next day for a biopsy. Yes! Now we were getting somewhere. I checked into the hospital. He was running a little early, so I got to show up a little early. But in true hospital style, somehow when the surgeon is running early, the time still stretches out between turnovers so that the case doesn't run that far ahead. In other words, it was hurry up and wait. I didn't mind. I know how it works; I have operated thousands of times. I was just glad to be there.

The surgeon came to see me in pre-op. He offered to do some mild local skin sedation with an injectable numbing agent, along with me breathing in some medication through a mask to make me sleepy and not care while he is doing it. That is referred to as IV sedation with mask general anesthesia. It typically does not involve any breathing tubes down your throat. He also thought that he would need a small incision. I thanked him for the offer, smiled sweetly, and said, "No doc. Just give me regular general anesthesia with intubation. I have a feeling that you are going to have more work to do than you think in there." He smiled and said okay. I finally went back to surgery. Everyone was wonderful. I woke up chatting. I was told that I was delightful. Apparently, they expect doctors to be assholes as patients. Well, I am glad I proved them wrong. The poor nurses were worried because I had so much swelling. They hadn't seen me pre-op to know that I was already swollen in the first place. I reassured them though. I also woke up with an incision that was at least four times the size he quoted. That didn't really surprise me either. He said it was a good idea that I chose general anesthesia. I was glad I chose general anesthesia too. Apparently, he told my husband that it was a matted mess in there. Well, I could have told him that! I got a little worried text from my oncologist later that night saying that it was especially important to start treatment as soon as the diagnosis was final. I was definitely on board with that! He was incredibly careful to say that, even though he was worried, he still felt strongly that whatever it is will be treatable. I appreciated that. Last thing I needed was to get my mental wheels spinning even harder while all hopped up on Norco. We still needed to get my port placed. It was supposed to be done while I was under at the same time as the biopsy, but some wires got crossed. I must admit that I was disappointed and frustrated to hear this. This was just what I asked before. Oh well. Nothing to do about it now. We will have to just get it scheduled.

CHAPTER NINE

BEST DAY EVER

ONCE AGAIN, the big wait was on. I was hoping for final results by Monday, but it was only Saturday. As fun as it was driving myself crazy thinking about the possible results, I had to find something else to do. I wanted to restart my daughter's horse lessons, which were two hours away and required us to trailer our own horse. It had been two months since we had been able to go. I know she was dying for a lesson. I was also dying to get back up there and do something kind of normal for a minute. Needless to say, the very idea seemed a bit daunting to the rest of the household. I had to do a lot of convincing that my little broken china doll self could handle it. After all, I didn't need to do anything except ride along right? No biggie. This also meant that they would have to do everything themselves with no help from me.

I finally got everyone on board with the idea, and we were off. It was incredible to watch everybody pull up their bootstraps and just get things done. They got the horse ready, got the trailer ready, loaded everything, and hitched up without me lifting a finger. It was both awesome and surreal at the same time. On one hand, it made me sad because I felt like a fragile guest observer at best. It gave me this weird glimpse into what it would be like if I weren't around. I tried to dismiss that thought quickly. On the other hand, I was proud of my family for just "getting it done." I knew the girls could handle it, but I was especially proud of my husband. My husband was never really an animal person, not because he didn't like them, but because he had had bad experiences and was afraid of them. Fast forward over twenty years of being married to me, and now we have a menagerie that includes large twelve-hundred-pound creatures that I know he is still afraid of even though he tries to hide it. It is kind of amazing that I still get to keep him.

We got all loaded up. I got all loaded up with my incision padding, ice packs, a travel neck pillow to keep my neck stable, plenty of water, lozenges for my sore post-intubation throat, and my buddy Norco, and we were off. Despite all the extras, I felt so happy and so normal. This was what we were supposed to be doing today! I was sure of it! All I had to do was sit and look out the window and enjoy. I was soaking up the sky, the scenery, and the company like I never had before. I wrapped myself up completely in the comfortable privilege of being there.

Two hours later, we arrived at the lesson, and it was like coming home. I had missed them so much! The trainers greeted us like we were family coming home for the holidays. It was wonderful. Of course, everybody went into full protect-the-china-doll mode and escorted me inside, gave me a chair, and propped me up with blankets. We also stopped to pray for me a minute, and they told me that their whole congregation was praying also. Wow! Unfortunately, I had to go and ruin it because I got woozy after daring to stand with my eyes closed for longer than a few seconds. They got all worried and then I felt embarrassed and started to cry so that just made it worse. It was a vicious cycle with me. I tried ridiculously hard to not have people worry about me and then when something happened and they did, I would cry which just made them worry more. Oh, for Chrissakes!

Once I was all settled, we got on with the lesson. I love watching my daughter work hard at something she loves. I love how she takes constructive criticism, and it just spurns her on more. It was a long three-hour lesson, and I loved every minute of it, just sitting and watching. I was sad to see it end, but I was completely exhausted, so it was time to go home.

The car ride home was a challenge, but I was determined to keep that to myself. My pain meds were wearing off. I tried to time my next dose, but the shaking of the truck had other plans for me. I kept quiet though. I didn't want to give them a reason to feel guilty or to prevent me from coming along next time.

I realized more and more just how important it is for cancer patients to have a touchstone of normality, despite everything that is going on. This is not just my stubborn side talking. Cancer patients have a need to participate whenever possible. I am not talking about doing things that are dangerous or could get in the way of our treatment. I am talking about staying involved enough in your life so that you still recognize it when you are all done with cancer. It helps us to keep going and to make sure that we keep in mind the hope that this cancer crap is temporary. The gut instinct of most family members of cancer patients is to immediately put the patient in a protective bubble to shield them from all harm. While sometimes this is necessary, most of the time it just leads to a sense of isolation and loss that can overpower a patient even more than the cancer can. I realize that it is more work to include them, depending on the scenario, but I'm tellin' ya ... do it anyway.

CHAPTER TEN

HERE COMES THE FOOD! OR WOULD MARIJUANA PLAY A ROLE HERE?

ONE OF THE benefits of having cancer is the food. Everybody assumes that you are not cooking regularly anymore because you feel like crap, so they want to help and drop off food. This was definitely true at my house. If I wasn't cooking, I am fairly sure that everyone starved or at least acted like they did. The food train did not last forever, but our porch became a daily repository of deliciousness for a while. Suddenly my family got gourmet meals every night! They were thrilled and I was grateful beyond belief. The irony was that I wasn't really thinking about food anymore because I was always nauseated and my appetite was gone, but I enjoyed watching them eat it. One night we had the most sublime and amazing Italian food brought to us with dessert, fresh lasagna, salad, and bread. We all sat at the table like we had just won the food lotto and dived in. I was full after about three bites, but I made myself eat anyway. Ugh, what a waste.

Of course, everybody noticed me not eating with relish. I confessed about my lack of appetite. Then before I knew it, I was getting expert advice on the benefits of marijuana from my daughter! What? How did she know so much? What the hell? Okay. I had to put that thought aside for a minute and just listen to her. My kids were trying to put me on drugs now? Marijuana? I spent way too much time discussing the realities and potential consequences of marijuana with my patients every day, and now I should consider it for myself? Did that make me a hypocrite? I mean, it would have been nice to have an appetite again. On the other hand, I am not really minding the weight loss without a struggle. I had never really been the person who got so depressed that they lost weight or got so stressed that they lost weight. Nope! Just the opposite. I packed it on like no one's business. This was the first time in my life that I was losing weight without trying. Yes. Yes. I understand that was not a healthy way to do it, but I was (and am still) a fluffy girl, and it's not like I didn't have some room to lose, ya know? I guess we had to table the marijuana discussion for now. I wasn't ready. In the end, I did not try marijuana, although everyone I met tried to convince me otherwise. I fully realize and embrace that it helps millions of people, but it didn't feel like the right choice for me. I was too uncomfortable with the thought of being even less in control of my brain and my thoughts. I was being forced to put enough foreign substances into my body already. I did not want to add another one.

CHAPTER ELEVEN

WAITING FOR THE PHONE TO RING

THE DAY finally arrived when my oncologist was supposed to call with my final results. The clock never ticked so slowly. It felt like I was waiting for an eternity. I remember the nurse pre call to prep me for his call. I now could answer yes to all the "bad questions" which I couldn't before. Well, that couldn't be good. She ended the call by saying, "You try to have a good day, honey, and good luck to you." OMG! What does she know that I don't? Yup. I started to panic a little. I started to cry. Why now? I already knew that I had cancer. I just didn't know if I had the "good one" or the aggressive one. I wasn't sure what my reaction was all about. I just needed to get that final diagnosis, tag my tangible enemy, and get started with this whole thing. However impatient I felt at the time, I needed to keep in mind that I wasn't even supposed to have my first biopsy for another couple weeks if we went according to the original timeline. I needed to be patient. Lord give me patience!

Finally, my oncologist called. He told me that it looks like

Hodgkin's. Hurray! BUT ... there was one stain that did not come out as expected, so they have to send my specimen to Mayo Clinic for a second opinion. Aw man! We were so close to the final answer. This meant that there would be another seven-day delay before we would know. Oh well. In the grand scheme of things, I was still further ahead on the timeline than I was supposed to be. I just can't do anything straightforward, I guess.

CHAPTER TWELVE

IT'S TIME FOR THE PORT

THE DAY of my port insertion finally came. I still didn't have the final pathology result yet, which made me a little nervous. However, it was a fairly sure bet that I was going to need the port, aside from a miracle from God or something. I didn't really see that happening. Something told me that I was supposed to go through all this so that I could use it to help patients later, and I was at peace with that. So, off I went to surgery.

I arrived at the surgery center with my usual flare and bravado, masking the rather intense anxiety that I was holding onto inside. I cracked jokes. I made people laugh. I fooled no one, least of all my body. The real me was discovered the second they took my ridiculously high blood pressure. Now let me tell you, even though I am a fluffy girl, I have always had relatively low blood pressure, which is a plus. Well, not today I didn't! Then they checked my blood sugar, which was also up. Ugh, I couldn't win! I felt like I was failing a test. Then, they had trouble getting my IV in, probably because I was dehydrated ... and the fact that I had already been accessed about a thousand times in the last month. I finally lost it and started weeping, not because I was in pain—I just suddenly had had enough. Then, everybody got all concerned and extra kind, which only made me cry more. I couldn't shut it off. I was trying desperately to switch back to bravado mode, but I just couldn't shift gears. I sobbed more, which only generated more concern and sympathy. It was a vicious cycle. Ugh. Finally, I calmed down right before it was time to go back to surgery.

Let's talk a bit about ports. First, why do you need one? The biggest reason is that it allows easy administration of chemo, fluids, and antibiotics without a bunch of extra needle sticks. It saves your veins for a rainy day after you are done having cancer. A port insertion is an interesting procedure too. In the procedure room, they give you a little "chill juice" so that you relax and do not care as much. You get a little oxygen, too, and a little IV sedation. Then they numb an area by your collarbone with local anesthesia and use a needle to access your subclavian vein. They thread a little hollow catheter into the vein and to your superior vena cava which is a large vein on the right side of your heart. They do this with the aid of X-ray technology called fluoroscopy. It's kind of scary cool when you think about it. Then they attach the port hub to that catheter, sew it in below your chest muscles, and close you back up again. Voila! Better vein access for all the meds and fluids you are going to need to get through this cancer thing. There are risks associated with it like damage to the blood vessels, infection, and blood clots. Fortunately, even though these are scary, they are relatively rare, and they do not outweigh the benefits of the port. Of course, it is up to you to keep the site clean and not do any swimming or hot tubs until your incision heals. Don't let your dog or cat lick it. This sounds like common sense, but you would be unpleasantly surprised at how often this happens. Honestly! You need to watch for redness or swelling or increased pain. Ports need to be flushed every time they are used or at least once a month to keep them from clotting off. Otherwise, they are relatively low maintenance.

Thank goodness my procedure went well, and I was significantly more chipper afterwards. I even took selfies with the nurses for my patient blog. Now I was ready. Bring on the chemo!

CHAPTER THIRTEEN

THE BEST THIRTY-FIVE MINUTES EVER!

ONE SATURDAY PRE-CHEMO I woke up feeling like a champ! I had slept a full ten hours ... without interruption! Holy crap! I didn't even feel like I had cancer! I had energy! I wanted to go kick some ass somewhere! I did a little dance. I told everybody in the house that I was ready to go. I sat down to breakfast thirty-five minutes later, smiling ear to ear. And then, without warning, it all started melting away. I felt the slow spread of heat and fatigue wash over me. I started getting short of breath and achy. I couldn't speak in full sentences without taking a breath. Within a few minutes, my cancer symptoms had swept back in, enveloping me in that blanket of sick that I had just swore I had shucked off for the day. Here I was again, the lymphoma patient, set up for yet another day on the couch. Aw man! One of the hardest parts, too, was watching my husband's temporarily hopeful facial expression slowly fade into the sad little empathetic smile that I came to know so frequently. This was, my friends, just the way it was. There was a level of unpredictability about this whole thing that was never easy to reconcile, much less accept. Welp, I guess it was time to dig out the remote again and settle in for some more Netflix.

CHAPTER FOURTEEN

THE FINAL DIAGNOSIS! OR HURRY UP AND WAIT

THE BIG DAY FINALLY ARRIVED. The Mayo Clinic second opinion was back. There were no more questions. I officially was diagnosed with the nodular sclerosing subtype of Hodgkin's lymphoma. Hurray! I *did* have the "good one!" This explains all the inflammation, the sweats, the weight loss, and the general ickiness. The sclerosing part meant that there were twisty inflamed bands of tissue coursing through the cancer cells, setting off additional inflammatory cytokines just to make you feel crappier. Okay, now that we knew for sure, it was time to get the chemo going right? Like yesterday? Nope. Now it was time to talk about possible clinical trials, repeating half the tests that I already had, and having to start from scratch to get specific chemo drugs approved by my insurance. More waiting. In addition, now that everybody finally decided that I did need a COVID vaccine after all, they wanted to wait until I got my second booster plus a week or so to even start chemo in the first place. So, there went another few weeks. I couldn't help but wonder, would this make a difference in my prognosis? Everybody said no, but I couldn't help worrying. I realize that oncology is not my specialty, but as a physician, I worried that every day without treatment is like a little ticking time bomb, one more opportunity for those cancer cells to get further away from you.

CHAPTER FIFTEEN

CONGRATULATIONS! YOU QUALIFY FOR A CLINICAL TRIAL!

HALLE-FRICKIN-LUJAH! A clinical trial! It's like the heavens opened up, and the rays of light are shining on you when you hear those words. It means that you have a shot at getting tomorrow's treatment today! It means that some of the meds will be "donated" in a way and not have to go through insurance. It also means that the treatment options are very likely less vicious with fewer side effects ... that they know of. You suddenly have access to experts from all over. Sounds amazing, doesn't it? There are some trade-offs though. There are thirty-nine-page consents with terrifying side effects to sign. You get assigned a navigator to help you get through it because now the process has become so complex that you need extra help wading through it. Your life transforms with a level of stricture and structure unlike anything you have ever experienced before. You have to dot every *i* and cross every *t* without fail, or you might get kicked off the trial. It is exciting and scary at the same time.

CHAPTER SIXTEEN

FINALLY, SOMETHING IS HAPPENING!

AFTER A COUPLE of weeks and what seemed like thousands of repeat tests, it was finally time to go to the oncologist's office and sign consents for the trial, get my first port flush, and do my chemo teaching. What a long morning that was! At first, I was so excited that things were finally moving and my chemo was finally approved. I'm thinking, *Let's go!* However, on the way in the car, my mind just started racing. I had already read the consent forms like a million times, and my brain was spinning with all the side effects and potentially terrible things that could happen ... in addition to killing the cancer. There were so many: heart arrythmias, low white blood cells, low platelets, bleeding, severe colitis, cardiomyopathy, severe infection, hair loss, just to name a few. It is pretty daunting if you think about it. The toxic chemo trade-offs seem like quite the price to pay to get rid of your cancer, but those are the options available at this point. Having said that, these effects aren't even as bad as effects from several years ago! Yikes! What were they then? Technology is getting better and better, and the drugs are getting even more specific and creative. I am grateful for that, but it is scary, nonetheless. Still, I was ready to move forward.

We went through all thirty-nine pages of the consent form and got everything signed. Then, it was time for the chemo teaching. The main nurse practitioner came in and introduced herself. She told us that she had been doing this for over forty years. Something about that felt instantly reassuring. In addition to the quoted years of experience, there was a way that she talked *with* you as a patient, not *at* you, that was comforting. It was like a mutual conversation with a friend who was willing to tell you like it is, give examples, and give you some idea of what to expect ahead. She also used humor in such a way that really resonated with me. For example, she knew that I was one of the main cooks in the family. As a result, one of the first things she told my husband was to kiss his gourmet dinners goodbye on chemo days unless he wanted to cook them himself because sometimes it just wasn't going to happen. When I was worried about getting too whiny or wimpy during chemo, she set me straight right away and said, "Honey! Are you kidding me right now? We just set off the equivalent of one hundred bombs and hammers in your body and expected you to tolerate it. You are not a wimp!" You see? She just had a way with words.

She explained how chemo would go and the timing of it. She went over side effects and what my options were for dealing with them. She explained about hair loss. I joked at the time that I was sick of my hair and more than ready for a hair do-over. I was chuckling on the outside, but inside I was not sure if I was ready to lose my hair. Hair loss is a big deal for a woman. Talk about a self-confidence crusher. I have already had problems with my hair in the past, but I have never had to deal with it falling out entirely. There is something about hair loss that is a real slap-in-your-face indicator that you are sick. When you lose your hair, you look sicker. There is no way around it. Every time you look in the mirror, despite wigs and scarves and disguises, you just know that you are undeniably sick. It gets hard to process.

As we continued to talk about chemo, I continued my tactic of laughing and joking on the outside to mask my anxiety on the inside. I am not entirely sure why I did that. Somehow it made me feel a little better to look like I was handling everything. I have this irrepressible need to reassure everyone else, sometimes to the exclusion of myself. I also just plain hate crying in public, and I am afraid that if I stop concentrating on reassuring everyone that I am okay, I will concentrate on myself too much and then the waterworks will flow. Sometimes I concentrate so hard on doing this, I forget to really listen to what the person is telling me. Fortunately, that day, I was able to strike a balance, and I was able to take in my instructions.

At the end of the teach, another nurse came in to flush my port. Let's go over what a port is again. A port is a silicone hub with an attached catheter that goes through the subclavian vein to the superior vena cava. It is usually placed under local and IV anesthesia with the aid of fluoroscopy to guide exact placement of the catheter tip. This little device gets flushed and accessed every four to eight weeks. It is a much better option for chemotherapy than your peripheral veins in your arms. The drugs can be so damaging that you wouldn't have any veins left to use later in life. So, how do they access it? First, they put topical numbing with lidocaine and prilocaine on your skin for ninety minutes or so. Then, the numbing is cleaned off with alcohol. A hollow Huber needle attached to a cartridge is used to pierce the skin and enter the hub of the port. The cartridge is attached to IV tubing so you can draw blood from it and give any kind of IV medication (like chemo) through it easily. The nurse was so fast it was over in a second. I could immediately taste and smell the saline. Blech.

We spent the next twenty minutes trying to plot out a schedule for the next six months of my life. We had to figure out chemo for several hours every two weeks, repeat lab sessions, intermittent CT and PET scans, and doctor visits. That was no easy task, but we got it done. Now to wait the last two weeks until chemo started.

CHAPTER SEVENTEEN

WE ARE ON OUR WAY ... OR ARE WE?

CHEMO TEACHING ... done.

Drugs ... ordered.

The rest of my life through June ... planned out.

Chemo start date ... in two weeks.

Okay we were on our way. What could go wrong now? We tried to find a balance between anticipation and fear leading up to the big day, not always successfully though. When the big day finally came, we gathered up our thoughtfully packed chemo entertainment bag and headed to the infusion center. Just as we were pulling into the parking lot, we got a call from the trial coordinator. Uh oh. That couldn't be good. Right? Well, maybe she was just calling to see if we were there yet? Maybe she was just checking on us? Nope! None of the above. She was calling to see if we got her email from last night. What email? I asked. The one that said your chemo did not arrive yet and that we were hoping it would come today. Whaaaaat? We were pulling into the parking lot and my medication was not there? My heart sank, and I felt

sick all at the same time. It was weird to have so much anticipation for something kind of awful and yet be disappointed
that it might not happen. What had my world come to? So,
we decided to go in anyway and at least get the doctor's visit
done and the labs drawn since we were already there. We
would wait until the morning shipment came. Maybe we
would get lucky. Unfortunately, two and a half hours later,
there was no luck to be had, and we had to pack up and leave
chemo-less anyway.

As we pulled away, the hope was that the chemo was
going to arrive in two days, and I could get my treatment
then. At face value it doesn't seem like that big a deal at first,
but it was a huge deal. That mix-up was about way more than
just a date change. It was a huge let down. I was all psyched
up to get treatment started. Plus, I had been taken off my
antidepressant because of possible drug interactions, so I was
dealing with all my feelings naked of any serotonin padding.
On top of that, in a matter of minutes, multiple schedules
were screwed up. My husband would now have to miss work.
I would have to miss more work. Delaying chemo for another
two days would mean that my goal of working the following
Monday was now a moot point because I would be in the full
throes of chemo side effects instead of two days safely past
them. This meant that I would once again disappoint a bunch
of patients and my staff, and I would be one step closer to
financial ruin.

Yes, I realize this all sounds overly dramatic, but it is all
true. I think that is one of the problems with this whole
system. Doctor's offices make decisions and say things, with
or without apology, and expect that to be enough to make it
up to the patient and send them on their way. In reality, it

isn't nearly enough. They need to stop and think about all the ripples of every decision. Communication is everything. They could have communicated with me before we arrived all the way down there. Here I was, all psyched up, about to embark on a potentially life-changing event, and it was ripped away. Of course, they didn't mean for it to happen, but the communication gap cost me just the same.

CHAPTER EIGHTEEN

THE BIG DAY

FEBRUARY 26, 2021 finally arrived. It was time to start chemo. This time, the treatment actually happened, but not without a few dozen more communication gaps that left me frustrated and upset, to the point that I had to call my doctor and ask/beg someone to please let me know without a doubt if my medication was going to be there before we got in the car and headed to the infusion center for nothing again. By four o'clock the day before chemo, I still hadn't heard anything, and I just needed to know. I was sure they thought I was hysterical and crazy, but I didn't care. Plus, remember, I was coming down off my antidepressants too. It really was a perfect storm. Ugh.

The treatment itself wasn't that bad. I think I was so glad to be getting started that I didn't care about the burning nose, red face, and bad taste in my mouth. I was getting chemo! I was on my way! I listened with a happy glow to the instructions that the nurse gave me before we left. I heard that I would probably have a great two days and then it would all come crumbling down after all the steroids and anti-nausea meds wore off. Okay sure. Sounds good.

My husband and I left the infusion center, pleasantly surprised at how I felt. It was dinner time, and I was actually hungry! I had not been significantly hungry in three months! It was time to eat. We went to a restaurant and had midday breakfast. I could have sworn that I died and went to Heaven. The influence of the steroids gave the food the taste of ambrosia, the likes of which had never touched my lips before. I ate the whole meal with relish. I could see my husband trying hard not to chuckle and smile as he watched me enjoy my meal. I felt so good! I felt like I could do anything! I had not felt like that in a long time. Then we got really crazy and went to the store and washed my car! I have to admit, the whole time I had a little nagging voice in the back of my head telling me not to overdo it, but I ignored it. I just wanted to enjoy the moment. The next day I felt even better! We even went for a walk!

And then, the next day happened ... the fateful third day they told me about. The feeling of ick crept up slowly throughout the day. By dinner time, I had to sit down halfway through making the food. I felt short of breath. My head was pounding. My sugars had gone wild from the steroids. My face was red. My body hurt. Oh man! Everything the nurse said was true! I am not sure why I doubted it or thought I would escape it. I was supposed to go to work tomorrow! How was that going to happen? I started to get anxious and pre-worried. I was worried this was going to happen when chemo got pushed back. The next morning, sure enough, I felt worse than death warmed over. Every step was a monumental effort. I just wanted to sleep. I had nausea and vomiting. My stomach converted overnight into a slowly emptying repository of rocks that felt awful. Every bite I tried to take just sat and went nowhere. My sugars were coming down but still bad, but I didn't feel like I had eaten enough to take my metformin. I needed to know if this was normal. I called the oncologist's office and left a message for the nurse. Several hours went by before she called, but when she did, it was just what I needed to hear. I laid it all out. I told her all the symptoms. I even confessed that I was worried that I was just some sort of wimp. She chuckled and said, "Are you kidding me? With the stuff that you got, this is all normal. You have to imagine that we just set off one hundred hammers and bombs inside your body with a slow detonator. That's why you feel like you do. You are *not* a wimp. Don't even think it. This is just you figuring out your pattern so that you can move forward from here." It was amazing to talk to her. It was just what I needed. It was reassuring. It was comforting. It was supportive. It made all the difference. It helped me get through.

CHAPTER NINETEEN

THE GUILT FACTOR

SO, now chemo had started. It should have been all smooth sailing from there, right? Wrong. You know, the further I travelled on the cancer path, the more I realized I really didn't know shit about all the things that come with cancer treatment: the side effects, the limitations, the financial ruin, the uncertainty, the relationship strain, the battles outside of the treatment room. But you know the one that really surprised me? The guilt factor! I didn't fully realize how *guilty* I would feel about being sick. I didn't really feel guilty about being sick, but I felt guilty about everything else: being a burden to my family, not being able to contribute as much financially, not being able to ease the worry of the people who cared about me, letting my patients down, inconveniencing everybody that had to help me with daily activities or transport, making things difficult for my staff. I just about made myself crazy over it. I had all kinds of people telling me to let it go and that no one could presume to tell me the perfect way to carry on with my treatment without inconveniencing anyone else unless they were actually in my proverbial shoes. I tried hard to listen, but that guilt held on to me like a ball and chain. It took me forever to make a dent in it, much less break it. It really got in the way of the healing process. It distracted me to the point of not being able to follow my doctor's guidelines sometimes. I found myself always pushing to do more or contribute more, which only made it harder for me to get well.

CHAPTER TWENTY

BUH-BYE HAIR!

MARCH 24, 2021—oh what a night! My hair was getting crappier and more brittle as the days went by, but on March 24th, we took things up a notch. My poor dog jumped up on my lap for a cuddle and wrapped her paw around my neck ... and came back with a paw full of hair. She promptly started panic-sneezing like Shih Tzus do and leapt off my lap only to look at me in terror with her paw still full of my hair. Needless to say, I had to extricate the hair from her paw. I ran my own fingers through my hair, and sure enough, the shedding had begun. Within minutes, I had shed enough that I felt fairly confident that the term *mange* could accurately describe my scalp at this time. It was time to take action! #baldmyway! I recruited my daughter Katy, and we headed for the bathroom mirror with clippers, scissors, razors, and shaving cream. We got the brilliant idea to make a Facebook video out of it, hoping to boost views and help me raise money for the Leukemia & Lymphoma Society. In the end, we had over 22,000 views, but no celebrity endorsements have come pouring in just yet. Here's the link if you ever want to check it out. I definitely give us points for creativity and enthusiasm. https://fb.watch/6u-m6p5THI/ We really did have fun doing it, and I think it helped people by showing them how to take an out-of-control, uncomfortable situation and make it on your terms as a patient. That really is the key with all this chemo stuff: find something amid all the chaos that you can have a say in or have control over. Sometimes that is the one thing that helps you get through that day. In addition, my kids informed me that my bald head did not look as disgusting as they thought it would. So, I had that going for me.

CHAPTER TWENTY-ONE

MOM, WHY DO YOU KEEP DOING ALL THOSE VIDEOS? YOU KNOW YOU DON'T HAVE TO

HONEY, I know I don't have to. I need to. I am an educator at heart, and I am always looking to help others. This was the perfect opportunity to do both. One thing this whole experience has taught me is that the level of communication and guidance for patients is lacking. I thought I could help change all that. Kind of like a cancer and chemo 101 course for patients. I started my I'm Gonna Lick Lymphoma Series on Facebook. I started making videos as soon as I started having symptoms and as soon as I went to my first doctor's appointment. I documented every treatment, every procedure, every feeling, what to expect, and how to handle bad news. I wanted to be the flashlight to light the way for other patients. I wanted to make up for the lack of instruction and the lack of communication for patients. Plus, it kind of redirected my mind and gave me new purpose while being sick.

CHAPTER TWENTY-TWO

HALFWAY THERE ... I HOPE!

APRIL 7, 2021 was the magical halfway point of my chemo-therapy. If all kept going according to plan, I would be halfway done with chemo after that treatment. Yay! The light at the end of the tunnel was coming into view. I trotted into the infusion center with a renewed sense of hope. I presented myself with a cheerful attitude even above and beyond what I usually armed myself with. Even the treatment went better than usual. No IV snafus or drug delays or anything. This time I wasn't going to get any steroids, so no more ridiculous and unpredictable emotional outbursts or sky-high sugars. Woo-hoo! The good news just kept on coming! Even when we had to go through the schedule with the follow-up scans and appointments, I was still floating on cloud nine. I even got out earlier than usual ... before noon! And, since we were on vacation, my husband didn't have to drop me like a hot potato at home and rush off to work. Awesome! We decided to head to our little cottage after chemo instead of home. It was a fantastic idea. I had missed it so much. That place gives me a sense of peace like no other. Just getting in the car to go there is like some sort of magical transformation in attitude. It was a good day.

This is a good time to talk about having a special or sacred space as a cancer patient. It is essential, as you are surrounded by chaos and decisions are out of your control, to find a place, whether it is physical or mental, to take a break. You need a spot of zen. You need something that is just yours, even if only for a moment. For some people, meditation is the key, a momentary mental separation and peace. For some people, it is a physical place. That place for me is our little cottage. It is on a hilltop on a small private lake, and I am telling you, complete transformation of mental state is possible there. There is nothing fancy about it. We have a little beach, a great view of the lake, and a little pontoon boat to put-put around in. It is my own little oasis. It calms me like no other place on this earth, no matter what is going on. It was and still is, absolutely essential to my ongoing recovery.

CHAPTER TWENTY-THREE

THE REPEAT SCANS ARE CLEAR!

NOW THAT WE had crossed the halfway point, it was time for another PET scan and a set of repeat CT scans. Yay! More radiation. This time I was really sweating because my sugars had gone wild with the chemo, and they had to be two hundred or less in order to get the PET scan. You see, with a PET scan, they inject you with radioactive glucose. The idea is that you fast at least four hours before the test so your cells are starving and hungry, especially the cancer ones. If your glucose is already elevated, there will be no incentive for the cancer cells to grab for the tracer glucose, and they won't light up. The PET scan itself is reevaluating your cancer status at the cellular level, looking for increased activity. The CT scan looks for actual tumors or gross disease. I was afraid that because my diabetes had been exceedingly difficult to control, I wouldn't be able to get my sugar below two hundred.

So, the CT scans came first. The radiology personnel were so amazing! They were actually excited to see me!

Apparently, they had been following me on social media already throughout my journey. That was so nice to hear. They also said immediately that they could visibly see that my neck tumor was smaller! Yes! Let it be true. My CT scans got done without a hitch and then came the wait. I knew that my doctors got the results within twenty-four hours, but no one called me. After a few days I couldn't take it anymore, and I called my doctor. He told me that my scans were clear! Halle-frickin-lujah! I was elated ... for about five seconds. The words hung in the air gloriously for a whole five seconds before he said, "But you know we still have to finish the trial treatment." Well duh! I know that! Have I given any indication that I was going to skip out on the rest? Couldn't I just enjoy the news longer than a few seconds before being reminded that I am not done yet? Please! I get it, he felt like he needed to be clear, but the timing was terrible.

On top of that, no one got around to scheduling my PET scan until it was almost too late. Someone forgot to tell someone to fill a prior authorization or something like that. All of a sudden, I was rushing to fit a PET scan in, missing work, and the only time they had for me was at 8:30 in the morning. I had to get up at 4:00 a.m., eat a mini meal, and take my insulin so I could follow the four-hour fasting rule so that I could have my sugar low enough to get the test. The same kind of pattern evolved with my PET scan results. Yay, they are clear, but you know you aren't done yet. Blah blah. Yes, I know. Seriously though docs, you have to give your patients a chance to absorb the rare, good news you have to give before you slam right into the bad.

CHAPTER TWENTY-FOUR

SO, MY CANCER IS GONE, BUT I STILL HAVE TO GET CHEMO?

BOY, life is just a little confusing and unfair sometimes. First you are on cloud nine because they tell you your cancer is gone, and then five seconds later you are reminded that you are *not* done with chemo. Then, on top of that, each chemo cycle seems to be getting a little more difficult than the one before. What the heck? No one has given me a very good explanation for this, but here are a couple of theories that seem to pan out. In one respect, it is like being a prize fighter. You keep getting hit over and over. Each time, your recovery is a little slower because you weren't fully recovered from the time before, and the injuries compound. Here's another one: the less cancer cells there are left in your body, the more the chemo is just attacking your normal tissue. Now, this one makes sense to me. I have definitely felt worse with each cycle. I have fewer and fewer good days when I feel like doing anything. I think I am down to four days out of every fourteen when I feel like a human capable of leaving the house. Yuck. But eye on the prize, I keep pushing forward!

CHAPTER TWENTY-FIVE

THE SEVENTH-INNING STRETCH

WOW, the morning of my seventh treatment I woke up on the wrong side of the bed. The two weeks after the sixth treatment had been rough with splitting headaches, intense joint pain, sweating and hot flashes, weight loss, neuropathy symptoms, and let's not forget the good old diarrhea that never ended. I was completely over it. I had a bad attitude. I just needed a revamp, and I wasn't sure I could do it myself. Wouldn't ya know it? I showed up to treatment, got all hooked up and my premeds going ... and then they told me I had to go home because my chemo wasn't even there! I had to go home! I can tell you right now, that this did nothing for my attitude. Not to mention it was the second time this kind of thing had happened. I was upset, depressed, and emotional, none of which made sense because I was dreading it anyway! Although, I think the extra emotions also came from the realization that lots of other people were going to be affected too: my patients, my family, and my staff. Everyone was going to be upset and struggling not to blame me for the inconvenience, but they still would be anyway. Oh, the guilt! I already spend too much time trying to make amends for things that I am not responsible for. This would be no exception.

But then, things turned around. Everyone buckled down and adjusted and did their jobs. I had time to do a lot of cleaning at home and tie up loose ends, and I got the opportunity to go to my little cottage and soak in all the nature and have a little bit of peace. Maybe that was meant to be.

CHAPTER TWENTY-SIX

ALMOST DONE ... OR ARE WE?

SO, here we are. The last chemo treatment is upon me, barring any more scheduling or shipping mishaps. The end is near. Just to say it out loud is really something; it doesn't even seem real. Could it really be true? Of course, when I speak in terms of the end, it really isn't the end. The next five years of my life will be well mapped out with follow-ups, appointments, and repeat scans and labs. "The end" doesn't really come until after those five years. There will always be that little forever shadow monkey on my back that things could take a turn for the ridiculous again, not to mention all the secondary cancers and diseases that can come from having chemo to treat the first cancer. Oh brother!

I would be lying if I said that I am not excited about the prospect of chemo being over. But, weirdly, at the same time, I am a bit terrified as well. No more chemo?! While that means, hopefully, no more of the awful side effects after they all wear off, it also means no more internal liquid defense system. It means that there could be more opportunities for the cancer to creep back into my life. Hmm. How will I know if it is coming back? In the interest of respecting the post-traumatic stress aspect of being a survivor, I made a promise to myself not to panic at every little twinge or symptom that I experience after treatment is over. But should I? Or should I be hypervigilant? This tactic saved my life before! I really don't know the right answer.

I am looking forward to feeling like myself again, to having stamina, to being able to exercise, to being able to have hair again (hopefully completely different and thick and amazing), and to feel, dare I say it, sexy again. But I hear that is going to be an additional wait as well. I have been told that it can take up to six months before patients feel back to baseline. This kind of statistic just makes me anxious because I suspect that it will be a natural tendency for everyone, including myself, to expect me to pick up right where I left off before treatment as far as work and life in general. I have a gift for putting extra pressure on myself, and I am sure this will be no different. Well, at least I am consistent in that regard!

Basically, what I am saying is that I am all over the place right now. I have no idea how to feel. Part of me is ready to throw caution to the wind and literally have a party (socially distant of course) to celebrate the end of this chapter. The other part of me realizes that there is a whole lot of other stuff to consider before the party can begin.

I think the biggest thing to keep in mind is to keep on keeping on. I don't need to know exactly what the future holds. I just need to hold on to the fact that there is going to be one. The rest will figure itself out.

THE CANCER JOURNEY
POEMS

A Change of Perspective/The Day After

I would swear today
My lump was a little smaller.
I could breathe a little better
And stand a little taller.
I took a walk outside,
Filled with joy, and nearly cried.
Maybe it's all in my head,
But I'll take that for now.
I'm letting go of my dread
And pushing forward somehow.
I thought of chemo as a punishment
For something I had done wrong.
But it's actually the path back to freedom
That I have unknowingly yearned for for so long.
2/27/21

The Choice

———

It's not a matter of loneliness.
It's the trade-off for the cure.
Waving at the window,
Staying home, secure.
Missing the parties and the hugs
And people that I love.
Looking forward to the bigger picture
Keeping my shiny new head above.
I will the target closer,
Lulling the finish line to my sight.
The reward for being good,
The win at the end of this fight.

3/13/21

The In-Between

———

Two weeks in between
Just long enough to forget.
Not long enough to enjoy it seems.
Not quite done yet.
Precious days of sun and normal appetite.
Enough to help me see
One day it will be alright.
3/21/21

Here We Go Again

———

Soaking up the last day
Making use of my energy
Before it ebbs away.
Relishing time in the sun
Before things get dark
And definitely less fun.
Feeling my faith and inner power
Determined to press on
Not letting thoughts go sour.
I can do this. I know I can.
Advocating for myself
This is all part of my plan.

3/23/21

Hope

───────

The sun spoke to her today.
It said, fear not.
There is time left to play.
There is time to run and strive and live.
There is time to feel and cherish and give.
There is time to shout out loud and say,
I will still thrive another day.
3/21/21

The Enemy Within

———

Microscopic soldiers
Out to destroy without permission.
Sly, clever,
Slipping through my defenses
Unnoticed at first.
I see you now.
I feel you now.
My battlements are in place.
The war cry has been called.
I now begin the process of your dishonorable discharge.
For now and forever.
The battle is mine to win
And win I shall.
3/23/21

Peace

———

Sitting in my favorite chair
Flames dancing in the air.
Reflecting back on my day.
Shooing any bad memories away.
Only quiet satisfaction remains.
Letting go of guilt sustains.
Allows my mind to rest.
Save myself for a bigger test.
3/29/21

Warriors

———

I looked around
And warriors were what I found.
Young and old
So many stories told.
Some long and some mercilessly short
No way to sustain their fort.
All with liquid weapons of choice
The only way to raise their voice
Against a mutual enemy within
Even as their strength waned thin
Still fighting in their own way,
Fighting to thrive another day
Pushing for themselves or a loved one
Until their battle is officially won.

4/4/21

No Wisdom Here

––––––

Sitting in chemo today
Listening to the chatter
Several elderly patients talking back and forth.
I eavesdropped a little, hoping to catch some wisdom.
Sadly, wisdom is not what I heard.
I heard anger, stubbornness, self-destruction, misperception.
"They can't tell me to quit smoking just because I have lung cancer!"
"I'll do what I want no matter what they say!"
"I've lived this long, haven't I? So why change now?"
My heart sank. No wisdom to gain here.
Lethal thought processes getting in the way of healing.
Confusing control with best interest.
Why were they here then?
Whose spot did they take?
Is there no gratitude for a potentially lifesaving option?
I quieted myself and my grateful heart.
Appreciating my doctors and nurses.
Celebrating my halfway point.
4/7/21

Who is That in the Mirror?

———

I'm a tired little warrior.
Too much out of my control.
But the fight fuels my fire
And is good for my soul.
I try to ignore all the other things
Like bloating, balding, and not wearing rings.
I tell myself it's okay
If I can't recognize my reflection today.
I'm still in there. I just need to see
That I have to go through this.
I have to do it for me.
4/8/21

Sometimes It's Hard

———

Sometimes it's hard
Hard to always smile
Hard to show good face
Hard to have a positive attitude
But you know what's harder?
Negativity
Frowns
Apathy
Each of those
More destructive than the last
Not for me I said
Not for me
I need all my strength
To fight the real enemy.
4/10/21

Private Cryin'

———

Secret tear
Dripping down my cheek
Reflecting what's inside.
Quick whoa!
Facade shield spontaneously raises.
Can't let anyone see that
Have to be strong
To help others believe
To help me believe
I can get through this.

4/18/21

I Forgot

———

Forgot what I was looking for
Forgot who I was looking for
A source of inner strength?
Secret cave of wonders?
A power source?
Something I was missing?
Hold on a sec
It's getting a little clearer
I don't need anything else
I don't need anyone to do this for me
I need to stop wasting time
Stop searching unnecessarily
I have what it takes
I can do this
4/18/21

Sometimes You Just Need to Cry

———

Hold on a minute
Close your eyes
Let the emotions rise and fall
Eyes watering
Heart pounding
Then open up the gates
Set it all free
Let it all go
Recharge from within
Regulate your breathing
Focus on a time
When you were happy, healthy
Excited for the next adventure
Allow solid, good memories to carry you
Lift you up gently when you can't support yourself
Rest your mind
Conserve your energy for another day
5/4/21

Almost There

———

It's not over yet, but we're close
Close enough to see the glimmer of light
Far enough away that we can't reach it
Liquid weapons pummeling the invisible enemy
Hit after hit
Like a prize fighter, I come back for more
Willingly and begrudgingly at the same time
Will to live is strong even though my body feels weak
The good days seem fewer and farther between
Ultimately it doesn't matter
Have to keep going
Have to show up
Have to represent
No one else can do it for me
5/4/21

Seventh-Inning Stretch

———

Cinco de Chemo
Actually Seis de Chemo
Like a seventh-inning stretch
So close and yet so far
I'm antsy even though I know it's necessary
Side effects more annoying
Emotions pouring out all over unchecked
Confusing my caregivers
I have trouble convincing them that it's okay, that I'm okay
I really do understand what's going on
I'm not falling apart or anything
Just a few crumbs breaking off here and there
just anxious to be complete me again
5/5/21

"The End" (When Chemo Is Complete)

———

We are almost there
Saying it out loud
Doesn't seem real
The real sigh of relief is five years from now
The shadow monkey on my back
Constant companion of what could be
Excited and terrified to be done
No more internal liquid defense system
Who will protect me? What will protect me?
Is hypervigilance the answer?
Or is living my life the answer?
It's probably somewhere in between
"The End" doesn't equal instant real me or whole me
Time, patience, perseverance is the key
Setting realistic expectations
That is the true challenge
6/7/21

Here are some links to my different video series and blogs:

www.facebook.com/laurakdoc
This is my office Facebook page and where the I'm Gonna Lick Lymphoma Series got started. Start looking in December 2020.

www.instagram.com/monroecomprehensivelasercenter
This is the Instagram for the office and our aesthetic center. It has a little bit of everything.

Laurakdoc.blog
This blog series is entitled Nothing's Off-Limits. We talk about a little bit of everything, except for politics!

Laurakatzmdpc.com
This is the main office web page. It goes over everything that we do.

www.podbean.com
Just look for "Straight Talk with Dr. Laura." This is basically the audio version of the blog.

www.facebook.com/groups/246607280530391/?ref+share-
This is the Facebook group I created called Chemo Peeps. It is a peer group for anyone ever affected by cancer or cancer treatment in which patients, family, and friends can have real one-on-one discussions about everything cancer and share tips and stories.

ABOUT THE AUTHOR

Dr. Laura A. Katz is a solo-obgyn in Monroe, MI where she lives with her husband and two daughters. She has been practicing medicine for over 20 years and has cared for women and girls of all ages with a wide range of health issues ranging from general ob care to cancer. She also owns a thriving aesthetic medicine business. She has made it her mission to care for and empower every woman she meets to live healthy and fulfilled, which is the same goal she sets for herself. When she is not practicing medicine, she actively volunteers with her local cancer support group, soaks up as much family time as possible, blogs, writes poetry, podcasts, and enjoys her garden.

CPSIA information can be obtained
at www.ICGtesting.com
Printed in the USA
BVHW031318160921
616891BV00004B/684